YOU AND
YOUR DOCTOR

YOU AND
YOUR DOCTOR

WHICH?
BOOKS

CONSUMERS' ASSOCIATION

Which? Books are commissioned and researched by
Consumers' Association and published by
Which? Ltd,
2 Marylebone Road, London NW1 4DF
Email address: books@which.net

Distributed by The Penguin Group:
Penguin Books Ltd, 27 Wrights Lane, London W8 5TZ

First edition October 1997
Copyright © 1997 Which? Ltd

British Library Cataloguing in Publication Data
A catalogue record for this book is available from the British
Library

ISBN 0 85202 690 0

You and Your Doctor contains information from several *Which?*
publications, including *Which? Way to Beat the System, The
Which? Guide to Complementary Medicine, Which? Medicine,
350 Legal Problems Solved* and *Health Which?* magazine, and
from the General Medical Council's *Duties of a Doctor*

For a full list of Which? books, please write to Which? Books,
Castlemead, Gascoyne Way, Hertford X, SG14 1LH
or access our website at http://www.which.net

Cartoons and cover illustration by David Pattison, Cartoon
Partnership
Cover design by Creation Communications
Typeset by Saxon Graphics Ltd, Derby
Printed and bound in Great Britain by Caledonian International
Book Manufacturers, Glasgow

CONTENTS

CONTENTS

INTRODUCTION

Choosing a family doctor, or general practitioner, is one of the most important health decisions you ever make. Yet most people do not give it much thought. And many people stay with a GP with whom they are not happy. As your first port of call for health matters, your GP is someone with whom you need to be able to communicate easily, and whom you can trust completely – not only with your own life, but with those of your family.

Most people change their GP only when they move house, registering with the one closest to their home rather than shopping around. But GPs vary enormously in their attitude to patients, their skills, knowledge and experience. If you have something specifically wrong with you – an allergy or mental health problem, for example – your doctor's attitude, experience and knowledge will have a big impact on the treatment you are offered.

Even if you seldom go to the doctor, you need to know that you can have an appointment when you need one, that you could talk to your GP if you wanted to, and that you would feel confident in your GP's care if you or any member of your family were to fall ill.

This book explains how the system works and how you can get the best out of your doctor/patient relationship.

GP PRACTICES

1

The GP (general practitioner) is an independent, self-employed doctor who has a contract with the health authority or board to provide services under the National Health Service. The UK has about 35,000 GPs. On average GPs have about 2,000 patients each on their lists, and it has been estimated that patients visit the GP about 4.4 times a year. About one-third of the UK's GPs are women (and half of those training to be a GP are women). The average age of the GP is falling: two-thirds are now under 50.

Most everyday diagnosis and treatment of patients is carried out by general practitioners, who occupy an important position in health care throughout the UK. The GP is the central figure in the 'primary care' team – the group of professionals from various health disciplines who work from a surgery or health centre. This team might include a district nurse, health visitor, practice nurse, community psychiatric nurse, chiropodist, therapists, social worker, receptionist and medical secretary.

The range of services that might be offered by or through a particular practice is extensive. It includes baby clinics, immunisations, child health surveillance, parentcraft, assisted conception, heart/blood pressure management, asthma clinics, diabetic clinics, family planning, cervical cytology (smear tests), well person clinics, health checks for new patients/older people, smoking clinics, diet/obesity clinics, dieticians' clinics, exercise advice clinics, stress clinics, minor surgery, cryotherapy (freezing treatment, often used for wart removal), phlebotomy (blood-testing), psychiatric services, counselling services, travel clinics (for holiday vaccinations etc.), chiropody, optical services, non-NHS examinations (for private medical check-ups), continence advice, minor injuries treatment, physiotherapy and speech therapy, plus complementary therapies such as osteopathy, homeopathy, hypnotherapy and acupuncture.

Many of these services, where available, are provided not by a GP but by a nurse or other health professional. If patients require any services not available within the practice, staff will be able to pass you on to the relevant provider, which will probably be the health authority or NHS community trust.

All practices now produce practice leaflets (see page 22) explaining what services they provide, in addition to other information, but some leaflets are very basic.

Doctors' duties

The first duty of any doctor is care of the patient. The General Medical Council, governing body of the medical profession, expects all doctors on its register to:

- treat every patient politely and considerately
- respect patients' dignity and privacy
- listen to patients and respect their view
- give patients information in a way that they can understand

- respect the rights of patients to be fully involved in decisions about their care
- keep their professional knowledge and skills up to date
- recognise the limits of their professional competence
- be honest and trustworthy
- respect and protect confidential information
- ensure that their personal beliefs do not prejudice their patients' care
- act quickly to protect patients from risk if they, as medical professionals, have good reason to believe that they or a colleague are not fit to practise
- not to abuse their position as doctors
- work with colleagues in ways that serve patients' interests best.

Doctors are expected never to discriminate against patients or colleagues and to be prepared to justify their actions to them.

How practices operate

Different doctors provide different services and facilities, and have different ways of running their practices. The advent of fundholding, whereby some GPs control their own budgets, has added another dimension of choice. In some areas patients of fundholders are likely to get quicker hospital care and more services than those of non-fundholders. Fundholding GPs have a budget for medicines, some hospital and other health care, and employing staff. A non-fundholder's bills are paid by the District Health Authority. Because they hold the purse-strings, fundholders have been able to negotiate better deals for their patients, and many GPs believe quicker hospital treatment is a major bonus of fundholding.

Fundholders are more likely than other GPs to offer counselling sessions, complementary medicine, self-help groups and specialist consultant clinics in their practice. Worries have been expressed about the two-tier system this could create, and about the time and money fundholding practices have to spend on accountancy.

Moreover, fundholders' practices may not be any better organised or be more accessible than others, and complaints about trouble getting an appointment and having to wait too long at the surgery are just as

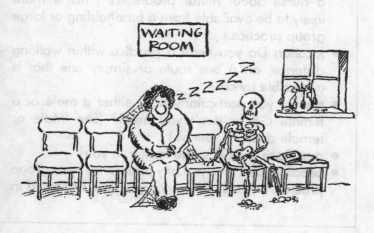

11

common in the fundholding environment as they are in other GP practices. So while it is as well to be aware of which sort of practice your GP runs, there are other considerations to bear in mind.

In due course the government will dismantle the competitive element of the 'internal market' in the NHS, bringing to an end the system which forces doctors, and indeed hospitals, to vie with each other for patients and funding.

What do you want from your GP?

- **services and staff** Do you want services such as counselling, health education and complementary therapies to be available? Would you value access to, for example, a well woman or family planning clinic? Would you like to be able to see a nurse about minor problems? (This is more likely to be available from a fundholding or large group practice.)
- **location** Do you need a practice within walking distance, on a bus route or simply one that is accessible by car?
- **sex** Do you particularly want either a male or a female GP, or don't you mind? (See 'Male or female doctor?', below.)
- **age** Does the GP's age matter to you?
- **practice size** Have you any preference for a group practice or for a GP working alone? The trend in

---

GPs' qualifications

A doctor who wants to be a GP does not take a specific examination in general practice. After qualifying as a doctor, trainee GPs do three years' postgraduate training, two in a hospital and one in general practice under an experienced GP. Most opt to take the entrance examination for membership of the Royal College of General Practitioners (leading to the MRCGP qualifica-

---

Britain is strongly towards group practices comprising four or more doctors. Note that although, at a group practice, you may have more choice, you may still face a long wait to see 'your' doctor.

- **opening hours** Do you want a walk-in surgery, fixed appointments or a mixture of both? Do you want an evening or weekend surgery? Do you need a mother-and-baby clinic, and is it at a convenient time? Do you want telephone access to your GP (or a nurse)?
- **approach/attitude** Do you want a GP who is sympathetic to complementary medicine, one who involves you in decisions, or one who decides what is best for you and then informs you of this?
- **special interests/expertise** Do you want a GP who has an interest in or knowledge of a specific condition, such as eczema or asthma?
- **facilities** Do you want a child-friendly practice? Do you need wheelchair access?

---

tion), but this is not essential. All doctors must be registered with the General Medical Council (GMC).

Special qualifications held by doctors include DRCOG (Diploma of the Royal College of Obstetricians and Gynaecologists), DCH (Diploma of Child Health), FPCert (Certificate of Family Planning) and DPM (Diploma in Psychological Medicine).

What makes one GP better than another?

A 1995 survey through *Which?* magazine established that what patients most want from their doctor is someone who:

- is prepared both to listen and to explain
- allows enough time for consultations
- keeps to appointment times
- stays up to date and involves patients in decisions
- provides adequate cover round the clock
- can get them the best and fastest hospital treatment.

The GP's ability to send you to the hospital that can treat you soonest is to a large extent determined by the complicated system of health-care purchase in operation as this book goes to press – ultimately a matter of government policy. So however much your doctor may wish to get you into hospital, his or her options may be limited.

All GP practices function better if patients themselves appreciate the time constraints. Try to be a responsible patient by cancelling appointments you cannot keep, making separate appointments for different members of the family and warning the receptionist if you are likely to need a little extra time.

Above all, however, it is the first point, about good communications, that is likely to be of greatest concern to you, and at long last the importance of doctor/patient communication is being recognised within the profession. Although it is such a major part of their job, some doctors do not find it easy to talk to patients. After all, their medical training has traditionally concentrated on the science and problem-solving aspects, not the human aspects (changes are being made, however: junior doctors now have to take an examination in communication with patients). Some GPs use a lot of jargon – or they talk down to us, or dismiss our concerns. Sometimes we find it difficult to understand, or remember, what we have been told, which may explain why about half of us fail to follow our GP's advice. If this sounds familiar to you, tell your GP about your concerns.

If English is not your first language and you have trouble understanding what your doctor is telling you, ask whether there is anyone available to help with translation and, if necessary, cultural concerns.

Sometimes the instructions given for taking medicines or other treatment are not easy to remember. It can help to take a few notes while you are in the consulting room – or even, if the doctor has no objection, to tape-record the conversation.

Male or female doctor?

Women doctors seem to be better communicators than their male counterparts, involving their patients in treatment options much more than male doctors, according to a 1995 study carried out at two London

15

hospitals and in Buckinghamshire.

Women doctors were found to be less likely than their male colleagues to ignore information volunteered by patients and to be better at encouraging their patients to talk. This applied whether the doctors were dealing with a male or a female patient, although women patients were found to fare even better than men. Male doctors also listen sympathetically to men but, the study found, are worse than their female colleagues at involving female patients in decisions about their health.

The researchers also suggested that male doctors tend to retreat behind a professional facade when faced with the 'socially threatening' prospect of dealing with women. As a result, they become much more 'medical' when dealing with women. Women doctors are generally better at helping patients to describe their symptoms.

Your doctor's willingness to involve you in your own treatment, and to listen to what you have to say, is ultimately of far greater importance than the male/female factor on its own. If you feel your doctor is not taking account of what you have to say, or you find him or her intimidating, and this concerns you, you may want to consider changing. Don't stay with a doctor you're not happy with, and don't wait until you are ill to find a new GP. Chapter 2 explains how to change doctors.

When your child is ill

Parents, especially if they are under stress, often seek home visits for their children, but in many cases there is no reason why the child cannot be taken to the doctor's surgery, especially if transport is available or can be arranged.

It can be difficult for parents to know whether a doctor is needed or not. Young children may not be able to describe what is wrong with them, their temperatures can fluctuate within a short space of time and they may seem ill at one moment but be perfectly all right an hour later. Pain can also be short-lived. In such cases, trust your instincts. If you think something is wrong, speak to the doctor.

When you should see your doctor

Although most of us have a pretty good idea of when we should see a doctor, it is possible to have something wrong without feeling ill. For example, if you notice any of the following, you should see your doctor within ten days:

- sudden weight loss (e.g. losing several pounds over a short period for no apparent reason)
- experiencing constant thirst, and hence the need to urinate much more often than usual
- feeling constantly tired for no apparent reason
- a change in a mole, breast or nipple
- a change in your voice, e.g. if it is husky or hoarse for more than three weeks
- frequent indigestion or belching
- loss of blood, e.g. from the stomach when coughing or vomiting, or from the vagina when urinating, or from the bowels.

If you have to take an ailing child to the surgery, telephone first, and warn the receptionist if you think the child is infectious. Once you are there, speak to the receptionist to minimise the delay between arrival and seeing the doctor.

You can probably arrange to sit in an area away from the other patients or to be seen at the beginning of the surgery if the child is likely to be infectious.

If you feel you are waiting an unreasonable length of time to see the doctor, speak to the receptionist.

Some parents worry about taking their child to the doctor unnecessarily. If you are seriously concerned, that is reason enough for taking him or her to the doctor and the vast majority of doctors and their staff will understand, even if the problem turns out to be insignificant. After all, many of them are parents themselves and know what it is like to be anxious about a sick child.

Out-of-hours cover

The vast majority of doctor/patient contact takes place within surgery hours, but emergency cover outside these hours is part of the NHS's commitment to the public under the Patient's Charter. Although you have the right to emergency treatment at any time, the rapidly increasing number of night calls (doctors receive five times as many now as they did 25 years ago) has forced GPs to try to rationalise the service. Some patients think nothing of ringing their doctors to demand an out-of-hours visit when the problem is very minor and could certainly wait until the next day.

There is however no definition of what constitutes an 'emergency' and if you have real cause for anxiety you should always seek advice by telephone (call the surgery first: the emergency phone number will be on an answerphone message), if only to put your mind at rest.

The rules of thumb are to ask yourself whether the matter could wait until the next day, and if it is a common ailment for which an over-the-counter remedy is likely to be available, try a chemist. For some problems, it may not be a doctor you need but a dentist, pharmacist, optician, health visitor, community nurse – or a midwife! In such cases direct contact with the practitioner concerned could be quicker and more effective.

To make the best use of resources while maintaining an effective service, many local GPs have set up primary care centres for out-of-hours treatment, or have formed co-operatives for this purpose. Fundholding practices in cities may use a commercial deputising service employing doctors specifically for night visits.

Out-of-hours emergencies

If you are faced with an emergency outside surgery hours, you will be able in the first instance to speak directly to a doctor and then:

- get advice on the phone
- be asked to visit the GP next day
- be asked to go to the primary care centre
- receive a home visit
- be referred to hospital.

If you have a deep wound that needs stitching, or think you have broken something, or believe your problem

19

cannot wait for a doctor to arrive (phone first for advice), go to your nearest accident and emergency (casualty) department.

Call an ambulance (999) if you or someone you are with cannot otherwise go or be taken to the hospital, or if you need a stretcher.

CHANGING DOCTORS

2

You do not have to give a reason for wanting to change your GP – although you may be asked. You are under no obligation even to tell your old GP. Just turn up at the new doctor's surgery, with your NHS medical card if you have it, and ask if you can be taken on. You will usually have some choice of GP, unless you live in a very remote area. If you live outside the area of your preferred GP you can still ask the practice to take you – it may be prepared to be flexible.

But you do not have an automatic right to be registered with the GP of your choice. GPs can choose not to take you (or to remove your from their list) without giving a reason. If the GP you choose says the practice list is full, there is little you can do. If, however, you suspect you have been refused for any other reason (for example, because you need expensive drugs, or because you are old), contact your health authority/board or Community Health Council (Local Health Council in Scotland, Health and Social Services Council in Northern Ireland), which you will find in the telephone directory. If you cannot find a GP to take you on, the health authority/board must do so on your behalf.

A GP can remove a patient from his or her list without having to give a reason. If this happens to you, the health authority/board will notify you, advise you to find another GP, and help you to do so. You will be entitled to receive treatment from your previous GP for eight days from the date of the letter telling you that you have been removed from that GP's list or until you have been accepted by another GP, whichever is the sooner.

Finding out about GP practices

Apart from asking friends and neighbours in your area, you can find out about local practices by asking for a list at the public library or the post office. Local pharmacists can be another useful source of information. You can also contact your local health authority or board, each of which publishes a directory of local GPs. Ask for details of practices which meet your criteria (for example, you might want one that is a group practice, or has a woman GP). Additionally, the health authority/board will be able to tell you the GPs' qualifications and when they qualified, practice size, what staff are employed, services available and languages spoken.

When you phone the practice(s) of your choice to ask questions (perhaps prompted by the subjects listed in the box on pages 12–13), take note of the receptionist's manner and attitude, which can tell you a lot. It is she who controls access to health staff and has the difficult and often unenviable job of trying to meet demands that all too often exceed resources.

Whether or not you are able to visit a few practices, do obtain the relevant practice leaflets. All GP practices must have one; it should tell you what area the practice covers, surgery hours, who works there, the appointment system, clinics provided, and arrangements for repeat prescriptions and emergency cover. This should help you to compare one practice with another.

Visiting GP practices

If you are able to make some visits to practices, look at the notice-board, pick up leaflets and get a general impression of each place. Is it a reasonably pleasant establishment in which to spend time? Do patients appear to be made welcome? Is there any privacy in the reception area? Are the staff helpful? Are there any toys for children to play with in the waiting room?

Some practices will let you have a pre-registration interview, so you have the chance to meet one of the

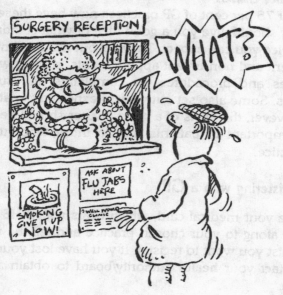

doctors (not necessarily the one to which you will be assigned) before finally deciding to register and judge his or her attitude, approach and communication skills. Not all doctors will offer such interviews – and, of course, they work both ways (the doctor will be able to vet you!).

If you cannot meet the GP, you may be able to talk to the practice manager: larger practices employ managers to control staff and services and deal with complaints, etc., to take the administrative burden off the GPs.

While you are there, ask whether the practice has a Charter.

Practice charters

Over 75 per cent of GP practices now have these, and they should give you a good idea of what standard of service you can expect. They set out waiting times for urgent and non-urgent appointments, surgery waiting times and procedures for complaints and suggestions. Some also set out what is expected of patients. However, the basis of a good charter should be what is important to patients, not to those who run the practice.

Registering with a GP

Take your medical card, which bears your NHS number, along to your chosen practice and tell the receptionist you want to register. If you have lost your card, contact your health authority/board to obtain a new one.

Once you have registered, the health authority/board will send you a new medical card and your medical records will be sent on to your new GP. Children under 16 need to be registered by their parents. Your children, or indeed your spouse or partner, do not have to be registered with the same GP as you. However, it can be helpful for a doctor to understand and treat a problem if he or she knows the whole family.

YOUR MEDICAL TREATMENT

3

Before you go to the surgery, think about what you need to tell your doctor. If your symptoms have been recurrent or been with you for a while, check the dates or number of occurrences. Consider whether what has been happening to you has affected your daily routine, and, if so, for how long. If you think you may need more time than is usually allowed for appointments, tell the receptionist when you book.

If you are taking medicines – including any you have bought yourself, such as herbal remedies – note down what they are.

If you have an idea about what might be wrong with you, tell your doctor. Also say what you would like to achieve, what you are afraid of and what you would like to know.

If you have already tried to remedy or ease the problem, perhaps after visiting another practitioner, tell your doctor this also.

Types of treatment

You have a right to know about your health and all aspects of treatment including any risks involved and any alternative treatment options. The NHS's Patient's Charter, launched in 1991 and extended several times since then, goes some way to close the information gap by explaining the rights and standards that you can expect throughout the NHS: it specifically states that patients must have their proposed treatment explained to them before being asked to consent to it. Having the right to know also confers responsibility on patients, so do use your doctor as a source of information and advice, and if questions are not answered to your satisfaction, ask for a second opinion.

For many medical problems, the standard form of treatment is a medicine, and in Chapter 4 you will find some of the questions you may wish to ask your doctor about what has been prescribed for you.

Stretched resources inevitably mean that the objectives of the Charter and the stated Standards are not always achieved. Some areas have more pressure on their budgets than others and doctors routinely have to prioritise, but this does not affect your rights as a patient.

Referrals

If you need treatment by a specialist, or the diagnosis cannot be confirmed, your GP may refer you to another practitioner. You can also ask to be referred, if, for example, you want a second (or third) opinion, but you will need your GP's agreement. For most NHS services, you will need a referral letter from your GP, although for certain types of treatment, such as physiotherapy, counselling or psychotherapy, you can refer yourself.

GPs can refer you for complementary therapies available on the NHS in your area (to find out what is available, contact your health authority or board and ask for the primary and community services section, which can explain how to contact the providers of the service).

You can also be referred outside your own area: fundholders are in theory able to refer you to any NHS

Your rights under the Patient's Charter

- to receive health care on the basis of clinical need, regardless of ability to pay
- to be registered with a GP
- to be able to change doctors easily and quickly
- to be offered a health check on first joining a doctor's list
- to receive emergency medical treatment at any time through a family practitioner, the emergency ambulance service and hospital accident and emergency departments
- to have appropriate drugs and medicines prescribed and to have any proposed treatment clearly explained to you, including any risks involved and any alternatives
- to be referred to a consultant acceptable to you when your GP thinks it necessary, and to be referred for a second opinion if you and the GP agree that this is desirable
- to have access to your (post-1991) health records, and to know that those working for the NHS are under a legal duty to keep their contents confidential

consultant or service provider who is willing to accept you; in practice, GPs often have their own contracts with particular hospitals and consultants and may need persuading to refer beyond these. Non-fundholders are limited by the contracts they have with the health

- to choose whether or not to take part in medical research or medical student training
- if aged between 16 and 74 and not seen by your doctor in the previous three years, to have the health check to which you are entitled under the existing health promotion arrangements; and to be offered an annual health check (at home if you wish) if 75 years old or over
- to be given detailed information about local family doctor services, including quality standards and waiting times, through your health authority/board's local directory
- to receive a copy of your doctor's practice leaflet, setting out the services he or she provides
- to receive a full and prompt reply to any complaints you make about NHS services
- to be guaranteed admission for virtually all treatments by a specific date no later than 18 months from the day when your consultant places you on a waiting list.

National Charter standards

Under this Charter, the NHS aims to provide the following standards:

- respect for privacy, dignity and religious and cultural beliefs
- arrangements to ensure that everyone, including those with special needs, can use the services
- information to relatives and friends about the progress of your treatment, subject, of course, to your wishes
- emergency ambulances that arrive within 8 minutes if the situation is 'life-threatening', otherwise 14 minutes in an urban area, 19 minutes in a rural area
- to be seen immediately and have your need for treatment assessed when you attend an accident and emergency department
- first outpatient appointments to be: 90 per cent within 13 weeks, the rest within 26 weeks
- to be given a specific appointment time for an outpatient clinic and be seen within 30 minutes of it
- waiting time for operations, including hip, knee and cataract surgery, to be no more than 18 months, and for coronary artery bypass grafts and associated procedures no more than 12 months

- not to have your operation cancelled on the day you are due to arrive in hospital (if, exceptionally, your operation is postponed, you should be admitted to hospital within one month of the cancelled operation)
- trolley waits (delay in admission to a ward from accident and emergency department) to be no longer than two hours
- a named qualified nurse, midwife or health visitor to be responsible for your nursing and midwifery care
- advance notification if you are to be admitted to a mixed-sex ward, with patient preferences for single-sex accommodation, including toilet and washing facilities, being respected wherever possible
- children to be cared for in a children's ward other than in exceptional circumstances, when a named consultant paediatrician should be responsible for the child's care
- hospital patients' dietary needs and preferences to be respected and a choice of dishes provided
- a decision to be made before you are discharged from hospital about any continuing health or social care needs
- patients receiving home visits from community nurses to be consulted about a convenient time and the visit to take place within a two-hour period around that time.

authority, and although they can request an 'extra-contractual referral' this will involve expense.

The Patient's Charter gives patients who are referred to hospital the right to see a consultant who is acceptable to them – for example, if you have a serious disease, you should be referred to an expert in the field. In practice, however, this often does not happen.

Questions to ask on being referred

- What exactly is the problem and why do I have it at this particular time?
- Why do you think I should see that kind of specialist, and that particular specialist? What is his/her experience in treating this condition/ doing this operation?
- What would happen if I chose to delay, or not to see the specialist?
- Is there anything I can do myself in the meantime to stablise or improve my condition?

Other sources of help

For many illnesses and disorders there now exist associations and support groups that can provide a form of help that complements what doctors do. However, doctors are not always aware that these exist or where to find them, and some may be reluctant to recommend a support group because many are an unknown quantity and the value to patients of what they do may be impossible to judge. It has also been suggested that some doctors have a over-protective attitude to their patients and do not want them to have access to information that might upset them.

However, it seems that most patients want as much extra information about their condition as possible and support groups are one way to get it.

Another possibility is to find out whether there is a complementary therapy that could help you. Some GPs know little about complementary medicine and are unlikely ever to recommend it to their patients, but in recent years many more of them have become interested in the subject and many now have complementary therapists attached to their practices. See Chapter 8.

Seeing a GP when you are away from home

If you are going to be away from home, say, on holiday or business, for a while (up to three months), you can ask a GP to accept you as a temporary resident. You can then be treated by the temporary GP should the need arise while remaining on the list of your home GP. You will not be issued with a medical card, nor will your medical records be transferred.

Again, if you have difficulty finding a GP who will accept you, contact your health authority/board for a list of GPs to approach. If you cannot find one who will accept you, the health authority/board will allocate you to one, and he or she will be obliged to accept you, at least on a temporary basis.

MEDICINES AND PRESCRIPTIONS 4

The most common form of treatment is a medicine, which can either be prescribed by your doctor or bought over the counter (many medicines are now available without a prescription, and indeed can cost less than a prescription). GPs will prescribe only a limited amount of a medicine at any one time – usually a month's supply – and many medicines have a limited shelf-life. So if your treatment is needed long-term you will need to get repeat prescriptions from your doctor (see page 38).

To improve the service your doctor gives you, and your own use of medicines:

- take an active part in understanding the illness and its treatment
- assume nothing
- ask questions
- become a full partner with your doctor in managing your illness.

Only you can feel and experience a painful condition or an illness, so try to be as accurate as you can in describing what is wrong with you or where it hurts and how long you have had the complaint. This will improve the accuracy of the doctor's diagnosis and choice of treatment.

Talking to a doctor about a health problem, particularly an intimate one, may be something you do not find easy. Doctors, too, can find it difficult to communicate with their patients, and time pressures can exacerbate this. Some doctors use prescriptions to avoid prolonging a conversation – or find that tearing the paper off the pad acts as a convenient signal for the patient to leave the consulting room. But if you are not sure why you are being given a prescription (or would like one but are not being given one), you should ask your GP to explain.

To help you obtain the information you want about any medicines described, a list of 20 questions is printed on pages 36–7. Try to get the answers to most of these, particularly in relation to medicines you take every day.

Keeping track

If you have to take a number of medicines daily and your doctor has not reviewed them recently, you should make an appointment so that they can be reassessed (this is especially important if you are over 65). Collect all the medicines, both prescribed and bought over the counter, that you are currently taking or have taken within the last month, and make a list of them as shown on the Medicine Record pages near the back of this book. Your local pharmacist will help you.

Many pharmacies can now hold 'patient medication records' – details of your medicines – on computer. If you go to the same pharmacy each time to have your prescriptions dispensed, the pharmacist can, with your permission, list the medicines you take on the pharmacy computer. Each time you have a prescription dispensed the pharmacist can look at your records to check dosages and directions and the risk of drug interactions. Some pharmacists will also record the over-the-counter medicines that you buy and alert you to any potential interactions with your prescribed medicines.

If your doctor has given you a prescription to take to the pharmacy, you may have to pay a prescription charge, but there are many exemptions. Also, it is worth remembering that now that so many more medicines are available without a prescription (in line with an EC directive that most medicines should be

---

Questions to ask about your prescription

Before the prescription is written

- Is there an alternative to treatment with medicines for my condition?
- How can I help myself apart from taking the medicine?
- What kind of medicine is it?
- How will it help me?
- How important is it to take this medicine?
- Is this a new medicine? If so, what advantages does it have over older products?

Before the consultation ends

- How and when should I take the medicine?

---

accessible to consumers unless there are specific reasons for restricting availability), buying the same product over the counter may be a cheaper option (see page 84). However, note that very few medicines are cheaper bought over the counter if you need large quantities for any length of time.

Where there are generic and branded versions of the same medicine, the generic one is likely to be the cheaper.

Prescription charges and exemptions

Those who are exempt from prescription charges are:

- How can I tell whether it is working?
- For how long should I take it?
- What may happen if I do not take it?
- What should I do if I miss a dose?
- Is the medicine likely to cause any unwanted effects? If so, how serious might they be?
- What should I do if unwanted effects occur?
- Will I need to see you again?
- What will you need to know from me then?

When the prescription is dispensed

- Can I take other medicines with it?
- Where should I keep it?
- Are there any foods or drinks I should avoid?
- Can I drive a car after taking the medicine?
- What should I do with any leftover medicine?

- men and women over 60
- children under 16
- students under 19 in full-time education

and, on production of an exemption certificate from the doctor or pharmacist:

- people on income support and family credit
- people receiving disability working allowance
- war pensioners, for prescriptions relating to war disablement
- pregnant women
- women who have had a child within the last year
- people with certain medical conditions that require continuous treatment, including diabetes, epilepsy, permanent stomas, myasthenia gravis, Addison's disease and thyroid conditions
- people with fistula (open hollow organ), such as colostomy or ileotomy, needing continuous surgical dressing or appliance.

No charge is made for contraceptive pills and related medicines such as spermicidal gels, creams and pessaries, or for devices such as the coil or diaphragm.

Repeat prescriptions

Prescriptions previously issued to a patient can be re-written without the doctor seeing the patient for another consultation. Surveys show that women and elderly people have a high proportion of repeat prescriptions, and that those most commonly issued without the patient being seen again are for medicines to treat rheumatic complaints, nervous and sleeping disorders, oral contraceptives and medicines for conditions that require long-term treatment, such as thyroid disease and high blood pressure.

If you need repeat prescriptions you can probably get a repeat prescription card from your GP listing the medicines you take regularly. You can give this to the receptionist for the repeat prescription to be written without your needing to see the doctor. However, this will take a day or so, so don't wait until you have run out of your previous batch to ask for the repeat prescription.

Repeat prescribing saves time and is certainly convenient for older people who cannot or may prefer not to travel to the surgery, or do not have a very good relationship with their GP, but each time a repeat prescription is issued an opportunity to review treatment is lost.

Although some diseases and their treatments may not change much over the years, the doctor is less likely to find out whether the medicine is acting properly, or whether adverse effects or interactions have occurred, if he or she relies on repeat prescribing. Repeat prescribing can also lead to medicines being continued for longer than necessary, and to over-subscribing. This can cause problems: for example, if you are prescribed antibiotics too often, they may cease to be effective; and if you are prescribed tranquillisers, you should take them only for a few days to get you through a crisis, not regard them as a permanent prop.

Information about your medicines

By 1999 all medicines must have a patient information leaflet included with them. Many already do, but sometimes the jargon and the poor design (especially the size of the print) make these less than user-friendly, which means that patients do not always understand why they are taking the medicine, how they should take it, what it is supposed to do, or what problems they could encounter (such as side-effects).

Most pharmaceutical firms do not test their leaflets on patients before publishing them, with the result that in some cases important warnings are not being heeded: for example, a 1996 survey revealed that six out of ten people suffering from asthma and half of those with high blood pressure had taken non-prescription medicines that they should have been warned to avoid.

The responsibility for getting the right information to the patient about medicines starts with the body that licenses the medicine, the Medicines Control Agency, which also licenses the patient information leaflet and the label or packaging in accordance with legal guidelines. When you are given a prescription, your doctor should make sure that the medicine is safe for you to take, that you know how to use it and what to do if there are any problems. The pharmacist should check this when dispensing your prescription.

For non-prescription medicines, safety checks should be made at the pharmacy before you buy them. The label and leaflet should make clear how to take it what the possible side-effects are.

40

The sorts of health risks from medicines of which patients need to be aware include, for example, symptoms being triggered in people with asthma if they take painkillers containing aspirin or ibuprofen: in this case, pharmacists should recommend a safer alternative, such as paracetamol. People with high blood presssure should avoid certain cough and cold remedies that contain decongestants, which could increase the risk of heart problems.

Doctors, pharmacists and patient information leaflets all have a responsibility to warn those with long-term medical disorders of the risks of taking certain types of medicine.

Taking medicines

- Always follow the directions on the label.
- Never take more than the recommended dose at the recommended intervals – taking more of a medicine will not make it work better or faster.
- Do not let anyone else take your medicine.
- Do not use medicines after their expiry date.
- Before giving a medicine to a child, check the dosage carefully; never give an adult dose unless directed to do so on the label.
- Do not give any medicines to babies of less than six months without the advice of a doctor or pharmacist.
- If you are taking a prescription medicine and want to take an over-the-counter product as well, check with your doctor or pharmacist first.

41

- To avoid choking, take tablets and capsules with plenty of water, sitting or standing upright.
- Swallow capsules whole unless you have been told to break them open.
- Liquid medicines are usually supplied with a 5ml spoon for measuring the dose. Syringes for measuring small quantities can be bought at a pharmacy or be supplied if the dosage is less than 5ml.
- If you find it difficult to open the container in which a medicine is supplied, ask your pharmacist to put it in a bottle with an ordinary top.

Storage of medicines

- Keep medicines out of the reach of children. Never leave any medicine lying around, even if you think it is out of reach. Do not let children play with empty medicine containers.
- Keep medicines in tightly closed containers.
- Do not transfer medicines from their original containers to other ones unless these are special medicine-reminder devices. Switching containers may cause you to lose the original instructions and may also affect the storage time of the product.
- Store medicines in a cool, dry place and protect them from light: a lockable medicine cabinet is ideal (unless there are special storage instructions such as refrigeration).
- Check the use-by date (expiry date), if applicable, on the label. Discard out-of-date medicines.

- If you have medicine left over once your treatment is finished, return it to your local pharmacy.

Disposing of medicines

Do not hoard medicines: take unwanted supplies to your hospital or local pharmacy. (Do not throw medicines in the dustbin or flush them down the toilet.)

Discard medicines when:

- tablets and capsules are two years old
- tablets are chipped, cracked or have changed colour
- capsules are hard and cracked or soft or stuck together

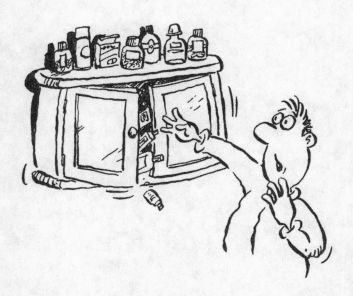

- aspirin and aspirin-containing medicines smell of vinegar
- ointments and creams smell or look different from the original
- liquids have thickened or discoloured, or their appearance or smell has altered
- ointment tubes are hard or have leaked or cracked.

DIET AND DOCTORS

The right food is vital for good health, and family doctors are required to promote health and to provide preventive health care as part of their conditions of service, so you might think that all general practitioners would be eager to encourage their patients to change to healthier diets. Diet, after all, is one of many factors that can affect your risk of certain diseases such as stroke, heart disease and some cancers.

Why diet matters

More and more research has suggested links between good nutrition and good health, from the protective effect of fibre (in fruit, vegetables, including baked beans, wholemeal bread and pasta, high-fibre breakfast cereals, etc.), to the anti-oxidant vitamins in fruit and vegetables. But few GPs have the time, knowledge or skills to give nutritional advice themselves, and not all practices employ dieticians or nurses with the right training to do it either. However, there has been a growing trend in recent years for people qualified to advise on diet to be available on-site.

Certain people can benefit in specific ways from following the right dietary advice.

If you are overweight, for example, you will know that this could contribute to a greater risk of heart disease, diabetes, breast cancer, high blood pressure, arthritis, back trouble and early death. You should be able to get some guidance on cutting down the fat (particularly saturated fat) and sugar you eat, and increasing your fibre intake.

Eating healthily does not in itself help you to lose weight: if you are eating too much healthy food and are overweight, you will need to reduce the amount.

Some vegetarians, too, could benefit from advice on how to avoid too much fat (cheese with everything is not the answer to a vegetarian diet!) while still getting enough minerals and vitamins, such as iron, calcium and vitamin B12.

For women who want to have a baby the recommendations are to avoid liver (because it contains high levels of vitamin A), raw or partly cooked eggs or egg dishes (including mayonnaise), soft-ripened cheeses such as brie and camembert, and pâté – all of which could cause infection. On the other hand, women planning a pregnancy should aim to have at least 600 mg of the B vitamin folic acid per day – which means eating leafy green vegetables and probably taking supplements as well. This will help guard against neural tube defects such as spina bifida in the baby.

Others who need specific dietary advice are those with high blood cholesterol, who could be at risk of heart disease. Correct advice should be available from all GPs' practices.

Getting advice on your diet

If you are concerned about your diet, start by talking to your doctor. Whether or not the GP suggests it, see the practice nurse as well, for a longer session where you can discuss the matter in more detail.

A health worker who is trained to help people change to a healthier diet – whether they are at risk or are healthy and wish to remain so – will ask you first about what you eat and how you feel about changing your diet: if you are not ready, no one can make you, and it may not be the right time in your life to think about such changes. If it is, you can discuss likes and dislikes and decide together on a few specific, simple goals – or maybe only one. Then you will agree on the ways in which you will keep track of progress.

If you have a condition with specific dietary requirements, ask to be referred to a dietician. You can see a dietician only if you have been referred by a doctor. If your GP will not do this and you would benefit medically from seeing a dietician, you have grounds for a complaint (contact the regional information service for your health authority/board for guidance).

PREGNANCY, MOTHERHOOD AND DOCTORS

6

To establish whether or not you may be pregnant, you can either use a pregnancy-testing kit (simple to use and highly accurate, these are available in chemists and supermarkets) or take a urine sample to your local chemist for testing. Alternatively, some GPs do pregnancy tests on their premises, or send the sample to a local hospital laboratory (there may be a charge for this service). All the tests look for the same hormone in the sample and give reliable results, unless the test has been performed too early and needs to be repeated a week or so later for this reason. However, a positive result will mean that the pregnancy is confirmed and you can start to plan for your baby's arrival.

Antenatal care

Pregnancy is dated from the first day of the last menstrual period and lasts approximately 40 weeks. During this time mothers-to-be undergo a programme of tests, scans and measurements and should pick up a lot of information about what is happening to themselves and their babies. Ideally, each woman should participate with her GP, midwife or hospital doctor (obstetrician) in deciding on a prenatal care plan.

Apart from preparing the mother and her partner for childbirth and parenting, this will focus on any problems that arise for the mother – such as heartburn, varicose veins and high blood pressure – and any signs that the baby may not be thriving in the womb. Mothers can expect about 15 medical checks during pregnancy and will also be given general advice on, for example, diet, smoking, exercise, alcohol and drugs.

As a pregnant mother you are entitled to free prescriptions and dental care while you are pregnant and for the first year of the baby's life.

Working while pregnant

About 75 per cent of women in paid employment continue to work until the 34th week of their pregnancy. Those with more than 26 weeks' service are entitled to 18 weeks' pay: six of these at 90 per cent of full pay and 12 at statutory maternity rate. Maternity leave can start as early as 11 weeks before the expected date of delivery; you will need a Mat B1 form to be signed by a doctor or midwife to confirm your expected delivery date.

Women now tend to work for as long as they can before the birth, provided they feel well and are not becoming over-tired (and the workplace itself is not hazardous), to allow for as much maternity leave as possible after the baby's arrival.

Maternity pay in the UK works out at an average of eight weeks' full pay.

Where to give birth

Conscious efforts, under the government's Changing Childbirth initiative, have been made in recent years to involve mothers-to-be much more in decisions relating to giving birth and to treating them as human beings rather than items to be order-processed in a factory.

The choice of where to have your baby is not a simple question of hospital or home. Certain other options offer some of the advantages of home birth but with emergency medical cover immediately to hand. Although the possibilities vary from region to region around the UK, the choices are:

- in hospital in a consultant unit
- in hospital in a GP unit
- under the 'domino' or district bed system
- at home.

'Domino' means 'domiciliary in–out'. Under this system antenatal care is provided by the community midwife, who becomes your medical minder throughout your pregnancy and in due course will go with you to hospital and deliver your baby. Unless problems have occurred, you can go home after about six hours, or, if your baby was born late in the evening, after a night's sleep.

If you want to have your baby at home, talk to your GP and your midwife early in your pregnancy. Most doctors are not in favour of home deliveries for the first baby because they cannot predict whether the birth will be easy or difficult. Although you have a right to a

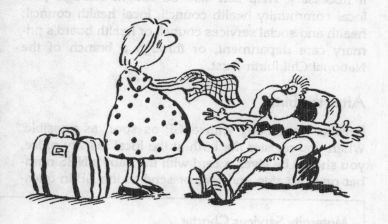

home birth, there may be risk factors (for example, existing conditions such as epilepsy or diabetes, a family history of high blood pressure, previous problems during labour, or known difficulties for the baby, such as an awkward position in the womb) which militate against it.

If your own GP is unwilling to take responsibility for you during pregnancy and home delivery and you feel strongly that you want a home birth, you may be able to register with another GP for antenatal, delivery and postnatal care while staying with your usual doctor for your other medical care.

If you cannot find a GP who is sympathetic to home births, or with recent experience of them, you should be able to book directly with your midwife, whose

51

responsibility it then becomes to find a doctor to cover if necessary. Help can also be sought through your local community health council, local health council, health and social services council or health board's primary care department, or through a branch of the National Childbirth Trust.

After the birth

Register your baby with a GP as soon as possible. When you register the birth at the local registry office, you should be given a card with the baby's NHS number on it, to sign and give or send to the GP in ques-

---

Maternity Services Charter

The part of the Patient's Charter dealing with maternity services sets out the rights and standards. It grants the mother:

- the right to choose where her baby is born (in hospital or at home)
- access to a named midwife who will be responsible for her care
- the opportunity to see a consultant obstetrician at least once during the pregnancy
- the opportunity to see a consultant paediatrician if the obstetrician anticipates problems with the baby
- the right to see her maternity records during preg-

---

tion. If the baby needs to be seen by the doctor before this card has been obtained, the doctor's surgery can provide a registration form. For babies, in particular, registration is very important because valuable time could otherwise be lost in the event of an emergency, so if you move house or go to live temporarily in another area make sure that you arrange for a local doctor to take you and the child on to his or her books.

Within a few days of your return home from hospital with your baby, you will receive a visit from the community midwife (you will already know her well if you had a home birth, and indeed she may have been present for it). The midwife will be available to you

---

nancy and, if she chooses, to keep them with her
- the right to be given information about local maternity services and an explanation of any treatment proposed, including benefits, risks and alternatives
- specific appointment times, and to be seen within 30 minutes of these times
- the choice of whether to have her partner or a friend or relative with her while she is in labour or giving birth
- the choice of having her baby with her in hospital — unless there are clinical reasons why she should not
- the right to have friends and relatives visit her in hospital at all reasonable times as long as this does not disturb others.

whenever you need her and usually has a 24-hour phone number to ring for help in an emergency.

The health visitor (who is also qualified nurse with special training in health promotion) will come to see you shortly after you arrive home, too – normally within about 10–14 days of the baby's birth. She will deal with any worries you have about the baby and also be available on the phone. She may be based at the doctor's surgery or local health centre, or at a child health clinic.

Checks on health and development, and immunisations, are carried out on infants at child health clinics, which are usually run by health visitors and doctors. Apart from providing the mother with a useful source of medical advice, these clinics can often provide formula milk and vitamins at lower prices than those on the high street and the contacts made there, especially with other mothers, can be invaluable. You will also be able to find out about support groups, childminders and very probably where to find second-hand baby clothes and equipment.

Going to Hospital

From time to time you may need to attend the outpatient department of your local hospital, because you have been referred by your GP to a consultation for examination, or to have hospital treatment that does not involve staying overnight, or for assessment and care in a nurse clinic. Alternatively, if you have been in hospital as an inpatient, you may have follow-up appointments.

Before you attend a consultant's outpatient clinic, you will be put on a waiting list; then the hospital will write to you with details of your outpatient appointment. The time spent on such waiting lists, and indeed the time patients spend waiting once they have arrived for their appointment, has often been the subject of complaint in the past and hospitals are trying to improve the situation.

The Patient's Charter now states that all patients should be seen in the outpatient clinic within 26 weeks of referral (and 9 out of 10 of them within 13 weeks); once you have arrived, you should be seen within 30 minutes of your appointment time.

Before hospital treatment

If you are about to go to hospital as an inpatient – say, for an operation – have a proper discussion with your GP about the procedure and the possibility of alternative treatment. It is also advisable to talk to the surgeon. If you are worried or feel you have not been given enough information, remember that you are entitled to ask for a second opinion.

Under the Patient's Charter, you should be given a written *and* a verbal explanation of what will happen during your hospital stay, before or at the time of admission.

Before any surgical procedure, or general anaesthesia, takes place, you will be asked to sign a consent form. (These are also used in the case of certain types of drug therapy.) First, be sure you have asked the following questions:

- what is the reason for the operation?
- what is going to be done and what are the risks?
- will I be treated by experts in the appropriate field of medicine or surgery?
- how long will I be in hospital?
- how long will it take me to recover?
- will I be in pain afterwards, and if so what pain relief will be available?
- are there likely to be any permanent after-effects?
- (if appropriate) will I be sterile after the operation, and will my sex life be affected?

Pain

It is always worth discussing beforehand with the surgeon how much pain an operation will involve, and finding out about the availability of painkillers. Some surgeons do this, in the outpatient clinic, and give patients a leaflet or booklet to read at home. Pain is not inevitable: modern surgical techniques have eliminated a great deal of post-operative pain. (See also below, under 'Pain following an operation'.)

Consent to treatment

No hospital treatment may be carried out without the patient's consent. If, having had the pros and cons of the proposed treatment explained by the doctor, you prefer not to have it, this decision will be recorded in your notes and must be respected. All mentally sound adults have the right to refuse to be examined or to be treated, and if this happens without consent the hospital could be charged with assault and battery – unless the patient has been detained under the Mental Health Act 1983 or has a notifiable disease. If the treatment carries any substantial risk or significant side-effect, consent should be given in writing. However, even consent given in writing will not be valid unless the patient has been informed about the treatment (including surgical procedures) and why it is to be carried out.

If the patient arrives at the hospital unconscious, the hospital will try to contact the next of kin to obtain consent for treatment on the patient's behalf. If delay would endanger the patient, doctors are allowed to administer any necessary treatment, but no more than is necessary to deal with the immediate crisis.

In the case of a child who is too young or otherwise unable to make his or her own decision, the law requires parents to give or refuse consent to treatment. Parents lose such rights (though they may be consulted) if the child is in care or has been made a ward of court.

Pain following an operation

If you are in hospital for an operation and are in pain afterwards, make sure the staff know this and ask for painkillers: remember that because different people have different pain thresholds it can be difficult for staff to know you are suffering pain, but you do not have to lie there accepting it. Do not worry about 'making a fuss' or 'bothering the nurse' (men in particular tend to adopt the stiff upper lip).

One way around the problem of being in pain while lying in hospital is pain relief that you control yourself, by pressing a button that administers a drug through an

---

The Children's Charter

Under this extension to the Patient's Charter, you as a parent can expect:

- your child to be cared for in a children's ward under the supervision of a consultant paediatrician
- your child to have a qualified, named children's nurse responsible for his or her nursing care
- to be able to stay in the hospital with your child
- (if your child is due to have surgery and where circumstances permit) to accompany your child into the anaesthetic room and be present until the child is asleep
- to be told what pain relief will be given to your child

---

intravenous drip – but there are still some patients who would rather adopt a stoical, grin-and-bear-it approach than make use of this facility.

Children in hospital

If your child goes into hospital, you should be able to stay with him or her as much as possible, including overnight, when the hospital should be able to provide a chair, mattress or folding bed for you; you should also have access to a toilet and washing facilities, use of a sitting room, kitchen, telephone and restaurant.

- the NHS to respect your child's privacy, dignity and religious or cultural beliefs
- your child to be offered a choice of children's menus
- to have breastfeeding facilities at the hospital
- your child to wear his or her own clothes and have personal possessions
- the hospital to be clean, safe and suitably furnished for children and young people
- all the staff you meet to wear name badges, both for security reasons and so that you know who they are
- your child to have the opportunity for play and to meet other children
- to have the right for your child to receive suitable education while in hospital.

Few hospitals now enforce strict visiting hours for parents, and many now keep basic food supplies (breakfast cereals, baked beans and so on) in the kitchens attached to children's wards for children who do not like hospital food. Most hospitals now let children wear their own clothes as much as possible, and to have their own toys.

Parents who are unable to stay with their children as much as they would like should let the ward sister know about any food preferences, habits etc. – even particular words used within the family – in order that she can make the hospital stay as happy as possible. All the nurses will have had some experience on children's (paediatric) wards, and some may have had specialist training in addition.

If the date for going to hospital has been pre-arranged, you should be able to arrange an advance visit to the ward with your child, which should help make the experience of the hospital stay less worrying. Books and leaflets have also been produced to help parents prepare children for going into hospital.

Leaving hospital

If you are being discharged from hospital, make sure you have all the information you need about dealing with any stitches and dressings, your medication, whether you can drive a car and how soon you can go back to work, etc. Find out whom to contact if any problems arise, and, if applicable, whether there are any support groups for your condition. If you need further medication, you will probably be given a letter for your GP explaining what treatment you have received.

Again, the Patient's Charter covers this aspect of health care. You, and if applicable (and with your agreement) your carers, will be consulted about your continuing health or social care needs before you leave the hospital, and decisions made accordingly. Under the Charter standards:

- you should be consulted at all times about plans for your discharge from hospital
- you should be given your own written copy of your discharge plan
- the hospital should make the necessary arrangements for any health and social care that you may need after you have left hospital
- you and your family should know what the after-care arrangements are
- your GP and anyone involved in your care should receive the information they need within 24 hours of your being discharged (for example, discharge date, diagnosis, treatment, ongoing support and so on)
- appropriate transport should be arranged for your return home
- you should not be discharged into a private nursing home at your own or your relatives' expense unless you have agreed to this: it is the health authority's responsibility to arrange this type of care if you require it.

Discharging yourself

You have the right to discharge yourself from hospital at any time, even against medical advice, unless you have a notifiable disease or are being treated under the Mental Health Act 1983 or have no one to look after you and are unable to look after yourself.

Provided you do not fall into any of these three categories you can leave at any time but may be asked to sign a form to say that you are no longer the responsibility of the consultant. You do not have to sign this. However, if you leave hospital against the consultant's advice and later need to be re-admitted the consultant could refuse to treat you: you would have to be referred to another consultant.

COMPLEMENTARY THERAPIES

Visits to complementary therapists exceed 4 million per year in the UK, and the number of therapists is increasing by 11 per cent per year, so there can be no doubt that interest in complementary medicine – also sometimes referred to as 'alternative' – is extremely popular. Surveys have shown that many GP fundholders would like complementary therapies to be available on the NHS, and four out of ten GPs already offer patients some form of complementary medicine.

Fundholding practices are more likely than others to offer complementary medicine to patients. Therapists can either be directly employed by the practice or, in the case of non-fundholders, engaged subject to the local health authority's agreement to pay for the service, or employed at a hospital, but clinical responsibility for patients remains with the GP. Some GPs are trained in one or more complementary therapies themselves.

The most commonly available therapies through GP practices are homeopathy, which uses minute diluted amounts of the substances that cause illness to cure its symptoms (the principle is similar to that of vaccination) and acupuncture, in which very fine needles are inserted into specific points in the body to relieve symptoms.

The appeal of complementary therapies to many members of the public seems to be that it can offer, assuming that an appropriate therapy is being used and that the therapist is competent:

- a good relationship with the practitioner, aided by the fact that there is likely to be less time pressure and often by the nature of the therapy itself
- a sense of personal control on the part of the patient
- an understandable explanation of the illness and treatment from the therapist
- effective treatment.

Availability on the NHS

It is not uncommon nowadays for acupuncture, osteopathy, chiropractic and homeopathy to be available on the NHS, while some hospitals use, for example, aromatherapy as an alternative to sleeping pills or to ease discomfort, acupuncture or massage for pain relief, and aromatherapy and touch therapies (such as reflexology) to alleviate stress. In these examples, the non-orthodox therapies are often used in conjunction with mainstream medicine.

Most reputable complementary practitioners who are not employed by the NHS are keen to work along-side conventional doctors. A complementary practitioner who advises patients to come off their prescribed medication is not to be trusted.

There are several homeopathic hospitals which take NHS referrals from GPs. Beyond this, the use of complementary medicine within hospitals depends to some extent on the interests and attitudes of the medical and nursing staff.

Finding a therapist

Whatever your reason for wanting to try complementary medicine, consult your GP before embarking upon any therapy and, equally important, be sure to liaise with him or her throughout your treatment. If your GP is unenthusiastic about complementary therapies as a whole, you are unlikely to get any useful recommendations on therapists. However, a local natural healing centre, if there is one, may be a good source of names of practitioners in your area and staff will probably be able to suggest which therapy would be appropriate for you. Natural healing centres usually have several therapists with different skills working in association with them. Word-of-mouth can sometimes be a good way of finding a reliable therapist but is far from infallible: what suits one person may not suit another, and just because your friend, relative or colleague has been able to form a good relationship with a therapist it does not mean you will.

Avoid picking a therapist simply from advertisements or mail-shots, or looking for one at a natural healing fair or festival.

Always check the practitioner's credentials before starting any treatment (or parting with any money).

The British Complementary Medicine Association or the Institute for Complementary Medicine may be able to offer advice on finding a competent practitioner.

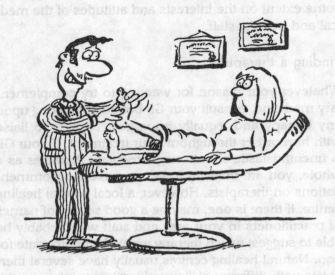

Therapists' qualifications

While doctors, nurses and some state-registered professionals such as dentists and physiotherapists must by law have received a certain amount of training before they can practise, most complementary therapies fall outside what medical schools teach and there are no government requirements for the training of complementary therapists other than osteopaths and chiropractors.

The situation is made further complicated by the fact that although many therapies have their own professional bodies (the British Homoeopathic Association is just one example), and a register of members, membership does not necessarily imply any level of training. Sometimes there is more than one organisation for a

66

single therapy, each of them claiming to register practitioners and often at loggerheads with the rival bodies. Many practitioners are not registered and for many therapies there is no consensus about the training needed prior to practising. Certificates or letters after a therapist's name might imply qualifications but could mean anything from a few days' training to years of it. Untrained or inadequately trained practitioners could cause patients harm or fail to notice a problem that needs to be brought to the attention of a conventional doctor.

Herbal and homeopathic remedies

All new medicines, under the Medicines Act of 1968, are required to be safe and effective before they can be licensed, but many of the older herbal remedies escape regulation because they pre-date the Act. Unlicensed preparations are thought to account for 8 out of 10 herbal sales and herbal medicines which are manufactured, sold or supplied by someone in a face-to-face transaction do not have to be licensed, although any which are potentially dangerous will be banned from sale by the government (comfrey, for example). Nor are herbalists required to list the ingredients in any remedy they provide, so it is advisable to exercise care and ask questions about such products, just as you would if your doctor were prescribing a medicine for you.

Note that although a product may be described on the label as 'natural', this description is no guarantee that it is safe.

CONFIDENTIALITY 9

Doctors must not disclose any personal information which they acquire during the course of treating you, unless you have given your permission. They have a duty to ensure that information about you is protected from unauthorised access while it is being stored, transmitted or received, or discarded.

When doctors wish to disclose information they must explain to patients what information this is, the reason for disclosure and the likely consequences. This applies, for example, whenever information is to be passed to others involved with your health care, and you have the right to withhold your permission. Information must be passed on in confidence.

Doctors must also respect requests by patients that information about them is not disclosed to third parties, save in exceptional circumstances, such as serious risk to the health or safety of others.

Conflicting obligations for the doctor

In the case of sexually transmitted diseases, and particularly HIV and AIDS, there may be a spouse or other sexual partner who is at risk, which puts the medical practitioner in a difficult position. The view of the doctors' governing body, the General Medical Council, is that grounds exist for disclosure to the partner only where there is a serious and identifiable risk to someone who, if not so informed, would be exposed to infection. A doctor with a patient infected in this way must discuss with him or her openly and honestly the implications of the condition, the need to secure the safety of others, the importance of continuing medical care and, importantly, the question of informing the sexual partner.

In the rare cases where a patient withholds consent to informing the partner, it is the doctor's duty to inform the partner in order to safeguard him or her from infection.

Access to your medical records

Under the Data Protection Act of 1984 you have the right of access to your computer-held health records from 1987. Under the Access to Health Records Act of 1990 you also have the right of access to manual files dating from 1 November 1991. (The Act in fact extends to records kept in the private medical service and Crown public service – prisons, armed forces, etc. – as well.) To gain access, you should apply in writing to the holder of the records in question (your GP or, in the case of hospital records, the health authority/board or NHS Trust). The application will state that you are the person to whom the record refers or are entitled to apply on this individual's behalf – for example, a parent in the case of a child, or a person managing the affairs of someone who is incapable of doing so on his or her own behalf.

If the record was made within 40 days of your making the application, access must be granted within 21 days. If the record is older than this the record-holder has 40 days in which to provide access. No charge is made if the record has been added to within the last 40 days, but if it is older than that a charge of £10 may be made. If you want a copy, photocopying and postage costs may be passed on to you.

If there are any terms in the record which are unintelligible to you as a lay person, you are entitled to have them explained, and to request changes if you find that the records are inaccurate.

The health practice or health authority/board holding the record is entitled to deny access to any part of it if, in its opinion, revelation would seriously harm the physical or mental health of the patient. Access can also be denied if harm could be caused to another individual or if the information relates to another identified individual who is not the patient or a health professional. Also, despite the legislation, it can be difficult to get access to records when you really need it. Make it clear that you know your rights, and be persistent.

CLINICAL TRIALS

In certain circumstances patients may take part in clinical trials without being aware that they are doing so: for example, they may be part of a control group of patients *not* receiving a particular drug being trialled. Generally, however, the necessity for consent to be obtained from patients participating in a clinical trial depends on whether the research can be expected to benefit the patient or not. If no benefit is expected, patients need to be given full information about the trial and to be able to withdraw at any stage. If the research is expected to be wholly beneficial, although consent should normally be sought, sometimes circumstances make it inappropriate – or even inhumane – to explain the details and seek consent (one such situation might be that of a patient who was fatally ill but did not wish to know this).

Your doctor might ask you to take part in a clinical trial if, for example, you have a heart condition for which a new drug is being developed; you may be asked to try it for a time to see whether you receive benefit from it. You are under no obligation to agree to participate in such trials, but if you would be interested in doing so you should be aware that safeguards exist:

- you have the right to know all about the trial beforehand and you should not agree to take part until you have had all your questions answered to your satisfaction, including all the known risks and the possible side-effects

- you have the right to withdraw from the trial at any time without giving a reason. You should not need to worry about repercussions affecting your future health care. (However, check beforehand whether pulling out of the trial early could have any adverse effect on your health)
- you should be allowed to see a copy of the results of the trial (but bear in mind that production of a research report can take several years)
- your case details and clinical data should remain confidential, but in practice this may not be possible since a pharmaceutical company monitor or official auditor may also be involved. If you are concerned about confidentiality tell your doctor that you would like your records to be seen by as few people as possible and made anonymous.

Among the questions you might like to put to your doctor before agreeing to proceed are:

- what is the purpose of the study?
- what will happen to the results of the research?
- may I have a copy of the results?
- what are the known risks and side-effects of the treatment?
- will I benefit from taking part in the trial?
- what can be done to help me if I have a problem while taking part?
- what will I have to do if I take part? Will there be lots of blood tests? Will I have to make lots of hospital visits or fill in many forms?

- will I be paid? Will the doctor be paid? If so, by whom and how much?
- has the trial been approved by a research ethics committee?
- why is the new medicine thought to be an effective alternative to existing treatments?
- may I have some time to think about whether to participate?
- may I have written details of the trial to take away with me?
- would I get compensation if things went wrong for me?
- what would happen if I changed my mind before the end of the trial? Would stopping in the middle cause any rebound effects?
- will I be able to continue taking the medicine after the end of the trail if I find it useful?
- will my heart be monitored after the trial and, if so, for how long?

All hospitals and other institutions where clinical trials are carried out have their own ethical committees to supervise the conduct of medical research.

COMPLAINTS ABOUT DOCTORS 11

Complaining is something many people find difficult, especially where human relationships are concerned. But it is not uncommon for breakdowns in communication to occur between GPs and their patients, giving rise to dissatisfaction, or for a patient to be unhappy about the treatment received or the fact that the doctor did not visit.

When such situations arise, it is important to be open and honest at the time about how you feel. Most people who complain want an apology, an explanation of why it happened, and to know that the same thing can be prevented from happening to others. Whatever the nature of your complaint, and whether the treatment received was through the NHS or the private sector, you should follow this sequence of action:

- in case there is a quick and easy way to have things put right, speak first to the person responsible to the treatment
- if you have tried but failed to resolve your complaint informally and decide to lodge a formal complaint, act quickly: delay could cause difficulties with evidence and may cause people to doubt how serious you are about your grievance
- keep copies of letters and other written records relating to your problem

- seek advice, whatever the stage you have reached with your complaint, from a Community Health Council (Local Health Council in Scotland, Health and Social Services Board in Northern Ireland), listed in the phone book, or other organisation or relevant pressure group
- be persistent, and be prepared for a procedure that is likely to be time-consuming as well as frustrating
- be clear in your own mind about the subject of the complaint (GP or other health professional), its substance (wrong kind of treatment, rude and uncaring behaviour, etc.), and the object of your complaint (what you want to achieve: an apology, a change of treatment, financial compensation, or simply to ensure that no one else has to put up with what happened to you).

Serious professional misconduct

Serious complaints relating to the professional conduct, attitude or behaviour of a doctor – for example, a major failure of care, unethical, violent or indecent behaviour, or dishonesty – should be made to the General Medical Council, which has powers to discipline all registered medical practitioners, whether in the NHS or the private sector. The Council can also deal with consistently poor performance.

NHS complaints

The NHS is a large and complex organisation and it can be difficult to know where to start if you experience

75

problems. The key features of the current complaints system are:

- rapid '**front-line response**' from the person responsible for the service concerned: under the quick, informal method of complaining direct to the provider of the service (or the practice's or health authority/board's complaints manager), the general practice or trust will respond to the complainant and endeavour to provide a satisfactory solution. It is intended that most complaints should be dealt with in this way, normally within 10 working days (20 if a health authority is involved)

- recourse to an **independent panel** if the complainant is still dissatisfied. The right to an independent review is not automatic but the review panel convenor will consider whether the matter is likely to be resolved in this way before taking a decision. The panel will comprise three members: the convenor, an independent lay chairperson and either another lay person (if the panel is set up by a health authority), or a health authority member or GP fundholder (if the panel is set up by a trust).

The sorts of complaint that might be dealt with by the procedure described above include delay in making, or failure to make, a house call, delayed or wrong diagnosis, delay in referring, or failure to refer, and poor treatment or communication. Complaints about family doctors or 'primary care practitioners' must be made no later than one year after the event that gave rise to the complaint (for dentists it is either six months after the end of the treatment in question or 13 weeks after you became aware of the cause, whichever is sooner).

Whatever your complaint, it is preferable to make it sooner rather than later.

Complaints about hospital treatment

If your complaint relates to hospital treatment, you should if possible start by telling someone close to the cause of your complaint (a doctor, nurse or receptionist, for example). If you prefer to speak to someone who has not been involved in your treatment, telephone or write to the NHS trust hospital's complaints manager, or general manager of the hospital or clinic, or the chief executive in the case of an NHS trust, and send a copy to the general manager of the health authority or board.

As well as your name, supply your date of birth or hospital number, quote the date of the incident, the names of the staff involved (or describe them if you do not know their names) and the main points of the case, stating clearly what you want investigated. Also state what you want to happen as a result – action by staff to sort out your problem, an apology, improved services for others, or perhaps an explanation (or more information) about what happened. If they would be relevant, ask to see your medical records.

Your complaint will be investigated by front-line trust staff and the Patient's Charter guarantees you a prompt response from the trust's chief executive (normally, this means a full response should be given within four weeks).

Most complaints are dealt with under this procedure, but if you are still not satisfied you can request a further review, which may mean that an independent review panel (see page 76, but also likely to include an independent clinical assessor) is set up. The panel will recommend what action should be taken to address the complaint.

Taking a complaint to the Health Service Commissioner

Patients may refer complaints to the Health Service Commissioner if they are dissatisfied with the NHS's response or if they disagree with the decision not to convene an independent panel.

Parliament has given the Health Service Commissioner (Ombudsman) broad powers to investigate complaints about NHS services. Being independent of both government and the NHS, the Commissioner can investigate cases involving clinical judgement and complaints about maladministration, staff attitudes, bad communication and inadequate handling of a complaint at source. To progress your complaint you will need to have evidence or to show that the service has failed you in some way, causing you suffering, injustice or hardship.

The Commissioner is likely to be the final resort once the two-stage complaints procedure described above has been exhausted and the patient is still dissatisfied with the response, or has had a request for an independent review panel refused. The Commissioner does not have to investigate every case brought to him (or her) but will exercise discretion before launching an investigation. Legal representation is rarely involved and the whole investigation will be confidential.

If you wish to take a complaint to the Commissioner:

- put it in writing, supported by any relevant documentation
- submit it within a year of the incident coming to notice: only exceptionally will a Commissioner waive the time limit
- either make the complaint yourself, as the person directly concerned, or ask someone suitable to represent you.

The Commissioner can obtain records and other documents from an NHS authority, and require its staff to give evidence, for the purposes of the investigation. The patient concerned, and, if appropriate, relatives and friends who witnessed the cause of the complaint, will be interviewed by one of the Commissioner's officers.

The findings are sent to the complainant and the individual or group under investigation. If your complaint is upheld, the NHS authority or trust may have to offer an apology, or change its policies or procedures to remedy any injustice or hardship it has caused. Very occasionally the Commissioner may recommend reimbursement of a financial loss that has come about through a failure identified by the investigation.

The work of the Health Service Commissioner is reviewed by a House of Commons Select Committee, which can require senior NHS staff to appear before it to discuss a case.

There is no appeal process for the Health Service Commissioner's judgements.

Note that the Commissioner will not investigate a complaint if you are also seeking financial redress through the courts (see below).

Seeking compensation through the courts

If you think you should be financially compensated for medical negligence, you do not have to have been through the clinical complaints procedure first, but obtaining compensation will almost certainly mean taking legal action, which you must start within three years of the incident that gave rise to the complaint. However, in the case of children, the three-year period does not begin until they are 18, so they have until they are 21 to bring proceedings. You can obtain guidance on pursuing the claim from your local community health council or AVMA (Action for Victims of Medical Accidents); the latter, as well as giving you free basic legal and medical advice, can refer you to a solicitor with the appropriate experience.

Claims for medical accident or negligence are not to be undertaken lightly, even if you qualify for legal aid. As well as being expensive, and likely to take a long time, such cases are extremely difficult to prove. Negligence is much more than a professional misjudgement. You will need a lawyer who is experienced in medical negligence cases, and having proved the existence of negligence your lawyer will have to show that this was the cause of your subsequent medical problems.

First, your solicitor will take a statement from you about what happened and discuss costs. If the matter seems worth pursuing, and you have the money to proceed or are eligible for legal aid, the solicitor will obtain the medical records, identify the issues and then send them to a medical expert prior to preparing a report. This will then be sent with your statement and records to a barrister for advice as to the strength of the claim and on how to proceed.

If your case is sufficiently strong, the health authority (or other defendant) may settle your claim out of court. If the case goes to court, it must do so within three years of the date of the incident or actions that gave rise to it.

Other avenues for complaints

Taking your complaint through the NHS procedure does not prohibit you from complaining to your local councillor or MP. For example, a maladministration complaint could be taken to your local government ombudsman. Forms for this purpose are available from council offices and Citizens Advice Bureaux, as well as from the local government ombudsman.

Complaints about private treatment

Whereas a serious NHS complaint could lead to your suing the hospital or the health authority, in the private sector you have to sue the practitioner personally because the doctor probably works independently, rather than being an employee of the private hospital or clinic where he or she works.

First, you have to establish that medical negligence or an accident occurred, or that a breach of contract occurred – or both. Your rights under the Supply of Goods and Services Act 1982 (common law in Scotland) are to receive a service that has been carried out with reasonable skill and care, within a 'reasonable time' where no time limit has been fixed, and for a 'reasonable charge' where no charge has been agreed in advance.

If you feel strongly that your private treatment was unsatisfactory you could initially withhold payment. Thereafter, you have the option of starting court action (see page 80, 'Seeking compensation through the courts', for where to obtain initial advice and how to proceed if you feel your case is strong enough to pursue).

If you are in a private insurance scheme you could ask the insurance company, before treatment starts, whether it is prepared to send the payment cheque to you rather than to the hospital or doctor concerned.

ADDRESSES

Action for Victims of Medical Accidents (AVMA)
Bank Chambers, 1 London Road,
Forest Hill, London SE23 3TP
0181–291 2793

British Complementary Medicine Association
9 Soar Lane, Leicester LE3 5DE
0116–242 5406

General Medical Council
172–202 Great Portland Street, London W1N 6JE
0171–580 7642

**Health Service Commissioner
(Ombudsman)**
England
11th Floor, Millbank Tower, Millbank, London SW1P 4QP
0171–217 4051
Wales
4th Floor, Pearl Assurance House, Greyfriars Road, Cardiff
CF1 3AG
01222–394621
Scotland
Ground Floor, 1 Atholl Place, Edinburgh EH3 8HP
0131–225 7465

The Help for Health Trust
Highcroft, Romsey Road, Winchester, Hants SO22 5DH
01962 849100

Institute for Complementary Medicine
PO Box 194, London SE16 1QZ
0171–237 5165

National Childbirth Trust
Alexandra House, Oldham Terrace, London W3 6NH
0181–992 8637

Which? Limited
Castlemead, Gascoyne Way, Hertford SG14 1LH
(freephone 0800 252 100 for book orders)
publishes, annually, *Cheaper than a Prescription,*
a booklet listing medicines which can be bought more
cheaply over the counter than for the cost of a prescription.
Price £2.99, p&p free.

INDEX

MEDICINE RECORD

YOUR NAME ....

DOCTOR'S NAME ....

DATE ....

ALLERGIES...............

Before you use the medicine

| Name of medicine | Date started | Why prescribed | How taken | | | How | Problems to watch for |
			Dose	Times per day	When	long for	

When you use the medicine

Name of medicine	How are you taking the medicine?	Any new problems?	Is the medicine working?

MEDICINE RECORD

YOUR NAME ....

DOCTOR'S NAME ....

DATE ....

ALLERGIES ....

Before you use the medicine

| Name of medicine | Date started | Why prescribed | Dose | How taken | | | Problems to watch for |
				Times per day	When	How long for	

When you use the medicine

Name of medicine	How are you taking the medicine?	Any new problems?	Is the medicine working?

MEDICINE RECORD

YOUR NAME ....

DOCTOR'S NAME ....

DATE ....

ALLERGIES...................................

Before you use the medicine

Name of medicine	Date started	Why prescribed	How taken			How		Problems to watch for
			Dose	Times per day	When	long for		

When you use the medicine

Name of medicine	How are you taking the medicine?	Any new problems?	Is the medicine working?

Here's just a flavour of some of the reports planned for future issues of *Which?*

- Multimedia PCs on test • Tumble driers • Stereo systems
- Compact cameras • Current accounts • Claiming on car insurance
- Health insurance • Shopping on the Internet • Washing machines
- Large family cars • Postal deliveries • Council Tax
- Package holidays • Credit reference agencies • Best Buy PEPs

So why not take up our trial offer today?

SUMMARY OF OFFER

3 free issues of Which? as they are published • Just fill in the delayed direct debiting instruction below and post it to Which?, FREEPOST, Hertford X, SG14 1YB • If you do not wish to continue beyond the free trial period simply write to us at the address above, and to your Bank/Building Society to cancel your direct debiting instruction, before the 1st payment is due • You first payment will be due on the 1st of the month 3 months after the date you sign the mandate (so for example, if you sign the mandate on 15th August, your 1st payment is due on 1st November) • No action is necessary if you wish to continue after the free trial. We will send you Which? each month for the current price of £14.75 a quarter, until you cancel or until we advise you of a change in price • We would give you at least 6 weeks notice in advance of any change in price, so you would have plenty of time to decide whether to continue – you are of course free to cancel at any time.

Offer subject to acceptance. Which? Ltd, Reg in England Reg No 677665. Reg Office 2 Marylebone Road, London NW1 4DF. Reg under the Data Protection Act. As result of responding to this offer, your name and address might be added to a mailing list. This could be used by ourselves (Which? Ltd, or our parent company Consumers' Association) or other companies for sending you offers in the future. If you prefer not to receive such offers, please write to Dept DNP3 at the above Hertford address or tick the box on the coupon if you only want to stop offers from other companies. You will not be sent any future offers for 5 years, in compliance with the British Code of Advertising and Sales Promotion.

--- ▼ DETACH HERE ▼ ---

Your name and address in BLOCK CAPITALS PLEASE

Name (Mr/Mrs/Miss/Ms)	Address
	Postcode

To: Which?, FREEPOST, Hertford X, SG14 1YB
Please send me the next 3 months' issues of Which? magazine as they appear. I understand that I am under no obligation – if I do not wish to continue after the 3 months' free trial, I can cancel my order before my first payment is due on the 1st of the month 3 months after the date I sign the mandate. But if I decide to continue I need do nothing – my subscription will bring me monthly Which? for the current price of £14.75 a quarter.

Direct Debiting Instruction Please pay Which? Ltd Direct Debits from the account detailed on this Instruction subject to the safeguards assured by The Direct Debit Guarantee. I understand that this Instruction may remain with Which? and if so, details will be passed electronically to any bank or building society.

Signed	Date

Bank/Building Society account in the name of	Name and address of your Bank/Building Society in BLOCK CAPITALS PLEASE

*Banks/Building Societies may decline to accept Direct Debits to certain types of account other than current accounts

*Bank/Building Society Acct. No.

Bank/Building Society Sort Code

To:

Tick here if you do not wish to receive promotional mailings from other companies □

Postcode

--- **NO STAMP NEEDED • SEND NO MONEY** ---